Poems on Nature
and Health

This edition published
by Little Oak Publishing 2024

@francoisehelenepoetry

Illustrations by
Colleen ODell,
Gordon Johnson
and StarGladeVintage

'Stay hopeful.' whispers
the sunset as its peacefulness
rest on my sorrowful heart.

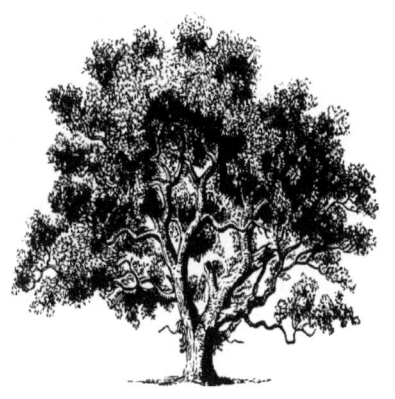

Children and Nature

As a child, nature was my primary source of entertainment. I used to spend hours cycling, and I remember, admiring the vibrant wildflowers and various shades of green from the leafy trees. The sea was my sanctuary, offering tranquillity for peaceful walks and escaping into my imagination.

In the Canadian winter, I'd skate on the ice rink in my backyard, paint the snow with my sister and brother, build igloos and spend lots of evenings on the swing stargazing.

Nature has always given me a profound sense of peace, and my love for it is unwavering today.

This poem, Remind Us, Children, portrays the everlasting calmness and playfulness that nature can bestow upon us.

Everyone should have access to nature, no matter where they are in the world. Without it, the wellbeing of the heart, body and mind may deeply suffocate.

Research shows that when children engage with nature, it improves their physical, social-emotional, mental health, cognition, wellbeing and increases resilience (1).

The importance of nature is not to be forgotten at any given time in our lives.

Children are especially good at reminding us that spending time in nature can be fun and valuable in various ways.

Remind Us, Children

Late afternoon. Children running
at the edge of the pines,
the fresh scent of mint looping laughs
in the eyes of children playing in the
evergreen wild.
If once again, you could be
behind those eyes,
you would see fluttering arms
against the silky blue sky -
plumed bird wings,
arches of resilient flights.

Descending swans rest
in open palms of freshwater lakes,
little hands reach up to greet
new raindrops from weeping clouds.
Young eyes in tired daylight
see currents of wonder in the empty
lives of sun-baked rivers.

Mornings unfold blankets
of brighter thoughts;
hopes for withered flowers to grow again.
A chance to roll down green hills,
down and down carpets by Earth rolled out
only for this, and octopus-branched
oak trees made for heedless,
happy falling.

Remind us, children,
of clouds of laughter
in winter's hoar breath,
the treasure of ripened conkers,
the taste of blackberries from grandma's
wicker basket hoard, the forgotten
music of tides reaching for coastlines
in the tender, restive air.

Remind us, children,
of Nature's richness—
stars, moon, mountains, seeds and sunsets.
With passing time, heartbeats slowdown,
but season to season, there always will be
beech, yew, ash and sycamore,
breathing with us, teaching us
the grace of breath.

Remind us, children:
this magical Earth,
brimming with living gifts,
timeless with wealth,
for all that's lost and past, holds us
cherished, still, and nurtures,
still, our health.

Veins and roots are all the same—
Children, remind us now and always,
how we live and die upon the soil
where growing hearts begin to play.

Illnesses and Nature

Researchers conducted a nine-year study at a suburban hospital in Pennsylvania, from 1972 to 1981(2). According to the report, patients with a window view of nature experienced quicker healing following surgery than those with a view of brick walls.

'Windows' is a compassionate poem exploring the potential for faster recovery and healing through exposure to nature, in contrast to a brick wall (2). It is important to note that although this theory was inspired by a specific illness in the research, it's extended to other illnesses, too.

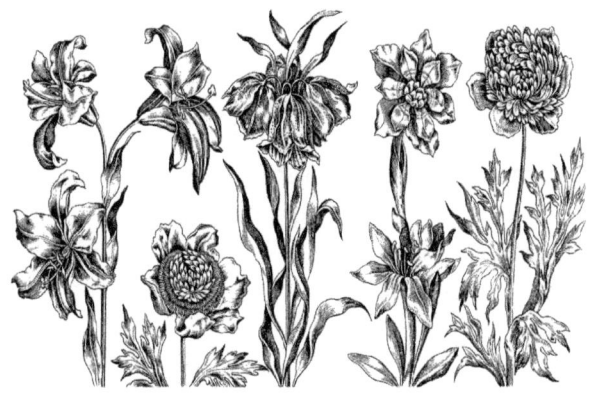

Windows

His lips tremble,
telling a memory;
soles bare, sinking in the damp earth,
each vertebra carrying
the core of his body.

He remembers, inhaling
the crisp air. The smell
of apples. The vibrance
of yellow decomposing
into amber. Shrivelled leaves
in the snow-white silence
of a new winter –
A quiet beauty, he saw.

The frame of life
now hospitalised.
Black thoughts spilled
on his memory's eyes.
Darkness stretched
across the breathless ward.
His body extends on a blank
canvas. In the room, a shut window,
a lifeless view. Only rigid bricks
to look at. Again,
they will not move.

The air trapped.
His lungs dry, very dry,
dry enough to make sowed
-skin suffocate. His heart
quiet. Cold in flesh.
His eyes drowsy
through a flash of death.
There is no more beauty left.

It isn't a lack of care.
It's this unearthly vision
that ties his soul into knots
and unveils an unobtainable tomorrow.
There is another world he must see –
one with trees growing
lines of oxygen.

Winter will come again
soon. Nature will look
sick like comforting death.
But in spring, green will revive.
The heart of dahlias will grow
while the hopeless bricks
fills with dust
like voided lives
in an unseeing silence.

Forest Bathing

Forest bathing, known as 'shinrin-yoku' in Japan, is an alternative medicine practice that boosts NK cells, aiding in illness prevention(3). It can lower blood pressure, reduce stress hormones, and aid in preventing depression, enhancing sleep, and promoting better moods(3).

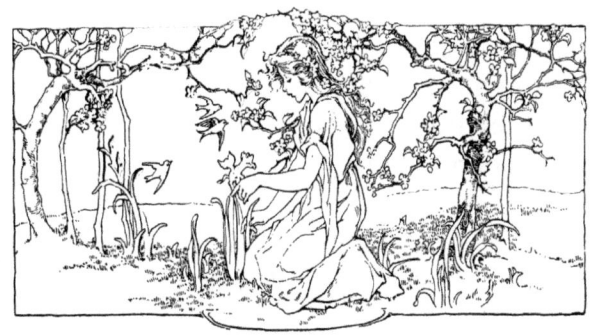

Forest

There is no sunlight,
only extended hours
in the office. On his way,
he loses his mind between
a maze of heavy traffic.

To his ear, a whisper reached -
words about a place in Japan.
With just a little time,
maybe he could find
sanity for his mind.
But to go, he must leave
his phone obsession behind.

Like a newborn, he arrives.
He gasps the cleansed air
and crawls with slow knees
in the depths of the forest.
His hands covered in dust,
he hauls the roots
of his carved pain.
Through the healing
of the earth, he holds
pieces of his worth.

The Pine's leafless branches,
tin as veins, entangled, clenched,
like anxiety in his body.

The rustling softens his screeches,
the wind, still.
His heart anew,
he listens to his own silence.

The rain washes over his being.
He's a young child again;
free of sins, deeply undamaged.
His soul, less broken.
In the mist, an outburst of
shameless tears. In his eyes -
a quiet sunlight breaks through.

Wellbeing and Nature

The Mental Health Foundation reports that individuals with a strong connection to nature live happier lives(4). Nature evokes positive emotions such as calmness, happiness and creativity. Nature encourages physical activity, which reduces the risk of cardiovascular diseases(4). Engagement with nature not only improves our general wellbeing but also improves cognitive function and brain activity(4).

I truly believe that it is critical for human beings to spend a lot of time in nature. Thus, we must cherish this time well spent. Connecting with nature helps us connect with our outer and inner worlds.

For Nature

For a day to rise in Australia
while the world sleeps in England.
For the earth to numb time
across distance to give
us more and more time.

For the sun to keep watch.
For its light to give way to the fields.
For withered plants
and summer roses to show
us how we feel.

For the blossom of echinacea
to carry hope we'll heal.
For winter nights help us see through
the soul's melancholic shield.

For the crackling of autumn branches
to echo in our bones. For their quiver
to remind us the mending
of our shatter is strong.

For the bird's voices to silence
rhythmic chaos in our minds.
For the heart to listen
and understand its own bounds.
For time in nature keeps
the heart and mind sound.

Humanity and Nature

The natural world seeks survival and growth. Beauty, destruction, and healing are all aspects of nature; within it, we find various species with similarities. Just as humans cannot live without a range of emotions, light and darkness are essential to nature.

This poem represents some foundations that connect us. None of us can live a life free of darkness. We sometimes hide and misunderstand the darkness within ourselves, yet it still resides within us. It's important to remember that we are not alone in our sufferings, as our paths often intersect with those of others, even though our experiences and pains differ.

Underground

In the hushed stream,
every fallen leaf, a folded heart.
Flesh heavy as stones,
the wounds creak at every drop.
Every ripple, a bleeding pain.

Dig, dig at the ground
of this cold, red water.
There are bloodlines
equally searching for
the roots of darkness
in the layered soil.

Look, there is buried grief
at every inch of this earth.
Pull the dead scabs
towards the light – for grief
only heals when it is seen.

About the author

Françoise Hélène is a Poet, Author, and Forest School Early Years Teacher. She's passionate about demonstrating how nature, art, literature, and music can enhance people's wellbeing. She also writes children's picture books and bedtime meditations and finds fulfilment in conducting occasional therapeutic poetry workshops for adults. She's a researcher who specialises in literature and wellbeing. She also enjoys writing song lyrics and has a particular fondness for singing in French, being her first language.

References

1.   Sharma-Brymer V, Bland D. (2016). Bringing Nature to Schools to Promote Children's Physical Activity. Sports Med. Jul;46(7):955-62. doi: 10.1007/s40279-016-0487-z. PMID: 26888647.

2.   Ulrich RS. (1984). View through a window may influence recovery from surgery. Science. 1984 Apr 27;224(4647):420-1. doi:10.1126/science.6143402. PMID: 6143402.

3.   Li Q. (2022). Effects of forest environment (Shinrin-yoku/Forest bathing) on health promotion and disease prevention -the Establishment of "Forest Medicine". Environ Health Prev Med. 27:43. doi: 10.1265/ehpm.22-00160. PMID: 36328581; PMCID: PMC9665958.

4.   The Mental Health Foundation. The Mental Health Foundation. Retrieved June 12th, 2024, from https://www.mentalhealth.org.uk/explore-mental-health/a-z-topics/nature-and-mental-health#:~:text=Research%20has%20shown%20that%20people,including%20lower%20depression%20and%20anxiety

5.   Jimenez MP, DeVille NV, Elliott EG, Schiff JE, Wilt GE, Hart JE, James P. (2021). Associations between Nature Exposure and Health: A Review of the Evidence. Int J Environ Res Public Health. Apr 30;18(9):4790. doi: 10.3390/ijerph18094790. PMID: 33946197; PMCID: PMC8125471.